I0408133

The Anti-Allergy Diet Guide with 34 Healthy Recipes plus a bonus a - 7 Day Anti-Allergy Diet Menu Plan

By Rebecca Publishing

The Anti-Allergy Diet Guide with 34 Healthy Recipes plus a bonus a - 7 Day Anti-Allergy Diet Menu Plan

By Rebecca Publishing

Disclaimer

All the material contained in this book is provided for informational and educational purposes only. No responsibility can be taken for any outcomes resulting from the use of this material.

While every attempt has been made to provide information that is both accurate and effective, the author does not assume any responsibility for the accuracy or use/misuse of this information.

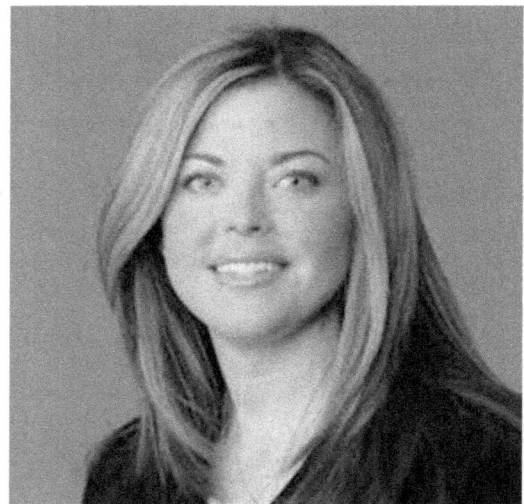

About the author!

I am a newbie to publishing business, but I have a lot of information to tell you. I have been studying healthy way of eating from leading nutritionist in Europe and I have a lot of useful information concerning this topic. I have lost more than 20 kilos so I can provide you with a lot of practical tips on this matter.

My story is also very bright, after giving birth to a child; I gained a lot of extra weight. It was simply impossible to look into the mirror, but I decided to do my best to return myself to my previous shape. I have tried swimming, jogging, different diets like Dukan, Sugar Free Diet, Kremlyovskaya Diet etc. These diets forced me to starving and nothing more. I saw and fell the best result after following the Paleo Diet combined with Ketogenic Diet. This diet helped me to loose ALL my extra weight this is more than 20 kilos/44 pounds and I feel myself much healthier now! I would like to provide you with detailed information about Ketogenic Diet in this book.

Table of Contents

Introduction

Thank you for downloading of my book The Anti-Allergy Diet Guide with 34 Healthy Recipes. If you wish to lose weight and stay healthy, like people say, to kill two birds with one stone, then this book is the proper thing for you. It gives you the clear explanation of what is anti-allergy diet, what is allergy, allergy symptoms, the causes of allergy, types of allergy, list of foods to avoid, list of food to eat and a bonus - 7 day menu plan for successful anti-allergy diet. To crown it all this book will provide you with 34 healthy and delicious types of recipes for successful diet. So lets begin our way to healthy life with beautiful body.

The Anti-Allergy Diet

Allergy is a disease of modernity, expressed in increased sensitivity to certain substances - allergens, that are contained in products, materials, air etc. Every year allergy affects an increasing number of people. Take a look around and you will see a lot of people with itchy red eyes, people who are sneezing, coughing and wiping their noses with a handkerchief.

What is Allergy?

In general, allergy is a reaction of people's immune system towards some kind of allergens. These substances or items generally do not harm the body system and functioning but sometimes body's immune system unknowingly attacks them and generate response. This response further causes some reactions in the body which in turn cause allergy. The human immune system rapidly reacts to these allergens and produces antibodies - special, natural filters that serve as a barrier to alien micro-organisms, many harmful and even poisonous substances. But when the filters are weak, their function is impaired or completely absent. As a result, all harmful factors begin their attack on the organs and tissues. Eventually, person starts to feel uncomfortable symptoms.

Allergy Symptoms

There are several types of Allergy Symptoms:

- common symptoms (fever, chills, lower blood pressure, disturbance of consciousness, pallor)

- local (coughing, tearing, sneezing, itching, dry skin, watery eyes, scratchy throat, red itchy eyes, nausea, diarrhea, rash, runny nose, rhinitis, dark circles under the eyes and others).

What should we do? How to get rid of unpleasant symptoms??? First of all, we rush to the pharmacy in search of salvation from unpleasant allergic symptoms, spend a lot of money on antihistamines which only improve our condition but not treat. Because in most cases, allergies are not treated. We go to doctors and try to find out the allergen that provokes symptoms and the cause of allergy. Scientists and doctors have identified several causes of allergies and allergic reactions. Here are they.

The Causes of Allergy

- sterile living conditions. We do cleaning using various household chemicals, which contains substances that kill natural bacteria. And the lack of some of them leads to a shift of the immune system and provokes allergic reactions.

- heredity (it is proved that allergy may be inherited from parents to children)

- diseases of the internal organs (stomach ulcers, nervous disorders, liver diseases etc.)

- environmental factors (pollutant emissions)

- frequent infections (especially among children)

Weeks passed, and we still suffer from allergies, the symptoms re-appear. What to do? You found out the cause of your allergy, you have strongly marked symptoms that cause a lot of inconvenience... there is nothing to do but to determine the type of your allergy.

Types of Allergy

Food allergy –it is provoked by different foods. The most allergenic products are milk (dairy products), eggs, wheat, soy, certain seeds, tree nuts etc.

Insect sting allergies – this type of allergy is caused by the bite of insects famous to cause allergic reactions such as redness, hives, pain, itching and swelling, etc. Beware of the honeybees, wasps, fire ants, hornets.

Skin allergy – widespread atopic dermatitis and Hives etc.

Dust allergy – this type of allergy is very dangerous and can provoke shortness of breath and tightness in chest, wheezing, asthma attacks, coughing etc.

Now, you know everything about allergy or almost everything. The most important question is still unanswered. How to save themselves? As allergy is an individual disease you should use individual treatment. To alleviate the condition of the body you may in two ways: with the help of medication, or take a Anti-Allergy Diet. This diet is the most effective way, irrespective of the type and severity of allergy, whether sudden or chronic.

Look into your fridge, think about what you eat... and the answer will not keep itself waiting long. Fast foods, fatty foods, smoked foods, sweets, dairy, allergic fruits, alcohol... and that's not the whole list of harmful products.

The Anti-Allergy Diet is a very difficult diet. Its aim is to eliminate from the diet foods with highly allergenic properties. This diet has both advantages and disadvantages.

Advantages:

The Anti-Allergy Diet helps to get rid of allergy and define the product causing the allergy. It helps to keep yourself in shape, gets you system back on track and lose weight.

Disadvantages:

It is very strict diet. A lot of products must be excluded from your daily diet. Duration - up to several months or more.

General principles of the Anti-Allergy Diet

In its composition this diet must be chemically gentle to the digestive organs and physiologically balanced to the body. It must contain the necessary amount of proteins, fats, carbohydrates and vitamins. In addition, it limits salt intake to 7 gr per day.

Chemical and energy composition of the Anti-Allergy Diet:

protein – 90gr, including animals

fats – 80gr with the animals

carbohydrates - 400 gr

the energy value is 2800 calories

Choosing this diet you have to make a point of using only right hypoallergenic products. Your motto should read as follows – Food is the best medicine!

The strict basic nutrition principles when you are on the Anti-Allergy Diet

Dietary Pattern

- eat fractionally 5-6 times a day. First, such a regime excludes overeating, which increases the load on the digestive tract, second, such type of nutrition helps allergic individuals to regain a healthy appetite, because many people lost it because of fear of allergic reactions.

Cooking

Food should be boiled or steamed. Roasting, baking and other types of cooking increase the content of different allergens in foods. At cooking chicken, fish or meat broths it is advisable to change the water three times.

Daily liquid use

You need to drink more water (about 2.5-3 liters per day), especially after meal. Liquid provides the output of the allergens and toxins from the body.

Alcohol.

It is clear that you must abstain from alcohol drinks (wine, port and beer, as they contain a lot of allergens).

Alcoholic beverages slow down the digestion and absorption of food and it is a direct way to the allergy.

Temperature condition

The optimum temperature of the food should be 15-60°C (not too hot or cold). Non-observance of temperature regime irritates the digestive tract and stimulates the nervous system, and any deviations from the norm may activate allergy.

The duration of the diet.

It is recommended to be on this diet for 2-3 weeks (for adults) and 7-10 days (for kids). The introduction of "dangerous" foods should occur every three days. It is necessary to monitor the body`s reaction. But if you decide to lead a healthy lifestyle and to get rid of allergies forever this diet should be an integral part of your everyday diet.

Fresh fruits and vegetables

Increase the consumption of fresh vegetables and fruits. They are rich in vitamins and fiber. Namely, the fiber helps to remove allergens from the body.

Ingredients for dishes

At cooking, you must follow simple recipes with minimal ingredients. Complex dishes make difficult to identify the allergen.

The variety of products

Don't focus on the same products. Use a variety of ingredients for your dishes!

And now let's see what foods are allowed and what are prohibited

Prohibited foods and why you must avoid them.

The main prohibited foods when you are on the Anti-Allergy Diet are animal proteins (milk, meat, fish, poultry). It is necessary to break a habit to use them or limit for some time. This is particularly true for fatty meat, milk or dairy products.

You should also avoid salty and smoked food (they contain large amounts of salt). Namely salt enhances the action of allergens. Semi manufactures, pickles, smoked meats, cakes and other products contain conservation and coloring agents which reinforce the manifestation of allergic reactions. You should avoid sour and spicy food: they irritate the stomach, disturb the digestion and provoke the aggravation of allergy. In addition, red vegetables and fruits are natural allergens.

Here is a List of Foods to Avoid

any caviar, seafood, fatty fish

milk, fat cheese, yogurts with flavors

eggs, particularly the yolks

different cheeses

smoked meat, sausages

pickled and canned foods, especially manufactured in an industrial environment

seasonings (pepper, mustard, horseradish, vinegar), sauces, ketchup

red and orange vegetables (tomatoes, beet, carrot, red bell pepper, radish)

fruits of the same color (raspberries, strawberries, red apples, melon, persimmon, grenades)

all citrus (the only exception is lemon)

dried fruits (apricots, raisins, dates)

mushrooms

caramel, chocolate, marmalade

coffee, cocoa, fizzy sugary drinks

honey, nuts

sour-crout

celery, sorrel

Allowed foods and why you must eat them

This list of allowed foods include only allergens-free products, that do not disturb the digestion.

To combat allergies, it is important to increase the consumption of foods rich in fiber and starch, which are digested in a neutral environment and do not irritate the stomach.

All products must be boiled or steamed. Thanks to this method of cooking, they retain nutrients and are easily digested.

Here is a List of Foods to Eat

dairy products (fermented baked milk, kefir, organic kind of yogurt without sugar and food dyes, low-fat cottage cheese)

lean beef, pork, chicken

lean fish (cod, sea bass, Alaska pollock)

offal (liver, tongue, kidney)

rice, buckwheat, corn breads

vegetables (cabbage, cauliflower and broccoli, green salad, fennel, spinach, parsnips, parsley, zucchini, turnips)

oatmeal, rice, barley and semolina porridges

vegetable oil, butter

green fruits (apples, white currant, gooseberry, white cherry, pear)

dried fruits (dried apples, prunes)

apple and pear stewed fruit and fruit drinks, green tea

still water

dry biscuits, lean bread

There are a great number of natural healthy means that support the human`s body and lower allergy symptoms.

VITAMIN RICH FOOD ITEMS

Vitamins are the most important ingredients for humans. Vitamins are the main enemies of allergy. There is a great variety of vitamins exist in the nature. Lots of them can help to treat the allergic reactions:

Vitamin C

Vitamin C is one of the most powerful vitamin which prevents allergic reactions. It is known that the histamine provokes allergy. This vitamin decreases the histamine production, strengthens the immunity of the body and combat against allergens. It is contained in such foods like oranges, lemon and lime etc.

Vitamin E:

Vitamin E is known as powerful anti-oxidant. The human immune system cannot "exist" without this vitamin because it improves the immunity. If people have strong immunity their body can easily combat against allergy. It is contained in such foods like spinach, tropical fruits, wheat etc.

Vitamin B15

Vitamin B15 helps to reduce muscular fatigue that is known to cause allergy. It is contained in such foods like seeds, yeast, pumpkin seeds, sesame and nuts.

Vitamin B5

If you are suffering from runny nose, sneezing (nasal and rhinitis allergies) you need this vitamin! It is contained in such foods like mushrooms, broccoli, liver, corn etc.

In addition, the anti-allergy foods enriched with vitamins reduce the use of drugs. Balanced, rational and healthy diet normalizes the work of gastrointestinal tract, increases the overall tone, nourishes your body with vitamins, helps to shed extra pounds and removes harmful decay products.

PROBIOTICS

Probiotics are microorganisms of normal intestinal microflora. What is their benefit? These microorganisms help to recover immune system of our body and lower the amount of bad bacteria.

If you will use foods with probiotics in your everyday diet, you will treat eczema, allergic rhinitis, asthma and food allergies.

Foods enriched with probiotics: yogurt (fresh organic yogurt without additives and sugar)

kefir (drink it twice a day on empty stomach)

BIOFLAVONOIDS

Bioflavonoids are substances of natural origin. It is nutrients-antioxidants, which is sometimes called "vitamin P". It is contained in such foods like green tea, red and yellow onions, apples, broccoli, raspberries, cherries, red wine and cranberries, etc.

FOODS ENRICHED WITH PHYTOCHEMICAL CURCUMIN

This phytochemical contains in turmeric. It has anti-inflammatory and anti-oxidant effect. Use dried or fresh turmeric in your diet. Add it in soups, vegetables and salads in moderate amount.

OMEGA-3

Omega-3 is a kind of fatty acids. It increases immune resistance. It helps to relief such allergic symptoms as cough, running nose, sneezing and improves the work of liver.

USE SPICES AND HERBS IN YOUR DIET

Spices benefit is known all over the world. Some spices help to treat allergy problems or relief its symptoms (eg. horseradish, hot mustard, fennel and anise). Herb and spices have anti-inflammatory effect which helps to lower the allergic impact.

7 Day Anti-Allergy Diet Menu

Recommendation: during the day drink more liquid – clean water, fruit or vegetable juice, any kind of fresh smoothie

The First Day (Monday)
Breakfast: cottage cheese with sour cream and sugar, tea.
Lunch: vegetable soup, a piece of boiled beef, green apple, yogurt.
Dinner: buckwheat porridge, steamed vegetables, pudding.

The Second Day (Tuesday)
Breakfast: oatmeal with butter and dried fruits, tea (green or black)
Lunch: vegetable soup, boiled pork, stewed fruit (or any juice you like).
Dinner: rice porridge, steamed chicken, yellow apple, yogurt.

The Third Day (Wednesday)
Breakfast: sandwich with cheese and butter, tea, yogurt.
Lunch: vegetable broth, a piece of beef, cucumber juice.
Dinner: mashed potatoes, boiled pork, banana.

The Fourth Day (Thursday)
Breakfast: boiled pasta with some butter, green tea, pear.
Lunch: vegetable soup with meat, stewed fruit.
Dinner: stewed vegetables, an apple, parsley juice.

The Fifth Day (Friday)
Breakfast: biscuits with butter, tea, banana and pear salad topped with yogurt.
Lunch: vegetable broth, steamed beef cutlet, banana, celery & spinach smoothie.
Dinner: buckwheat porridge with steamed vegetables, tea.

The Sixth Day (Saturday)
Breakfast: law-fat cottage cheese casserole, Pineapple Kale Cucumber raw juice.
Lunch: vegetable broth, a piece of boiled beef, stewed fruits.
Dinner: rice porridge, yoghurt, banana.

The Seventh Day (Sunday)
Breakfast: bread with butter and boiled meat, one yellow pear, black tea.
Lunch: vegetable soup, steamed chicken, one banana, green smoothie.
Dinner: porridge, vegetable salad with herbs, yogurt.

ANTI-ALLERGY RECIPES

<u>Anti-Allergy Beverages</u>

1. Anti-Allergy Raw Juice

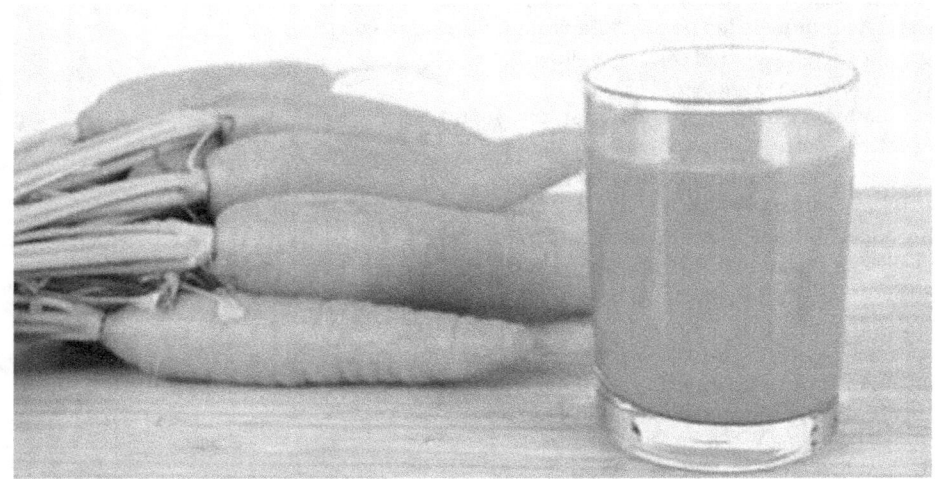

INGREDIENTS:

Red radish – 1 piece
Garlic bulbets – 1 piece
Half of one small red onion
Carrot - 1 piece
Pear - 1 piece
Cabbage leaves -2 pcs

DIRECTIONS:

1. Wash, peel (if necessary) and chop all ingredients.
2. Make a fresh raw juice with a juicer.

<u>Tips and Tricks:</u> Add ice cubes or dilute with filtered water or cold herbal tea (if necessary).

Drink 250-300 ml of your favorite raw juice daily.

2. Simple Green Juice

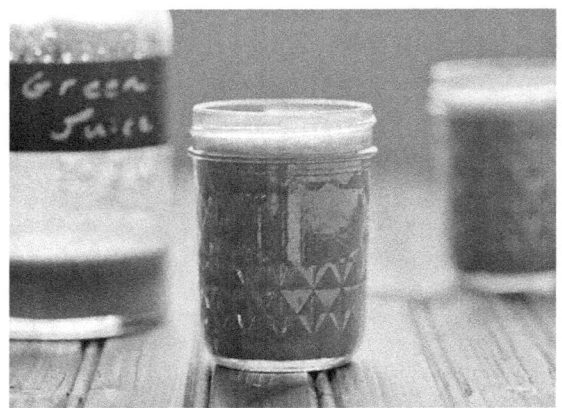

INGREDIENTS:

Half of one cucumber
Celery stalks – 3 pcs
Spinach – 150 g (chopped)
Kale leaves – 3 pcs
Half of one lemon
Apples – 2 pcs

DIRECTIONS:

1. Wash, peel (if necessary) and chop all ingredients.
2. Put all ingredients in your juicer and make a fresh green juice.

3. Green Detox

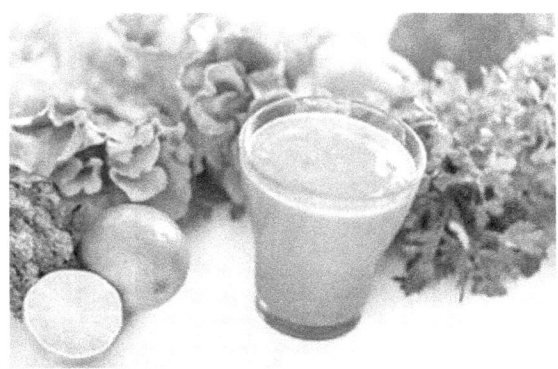

INGREDIENTS:

Half of one Romaine lettuce head
Spinach -30 g (chopped)
Kale leaves – 2 pcs
Cilantro - 10 sprigs
Apples – 2 pcs
Half of one lime

DIRECTIONS:

1. Wash, peel (if necessary) and chop all ingredients.
2. Put all ingredients in your juicer and make a fresh green juice.

4. Pineapple Kale Cucumber

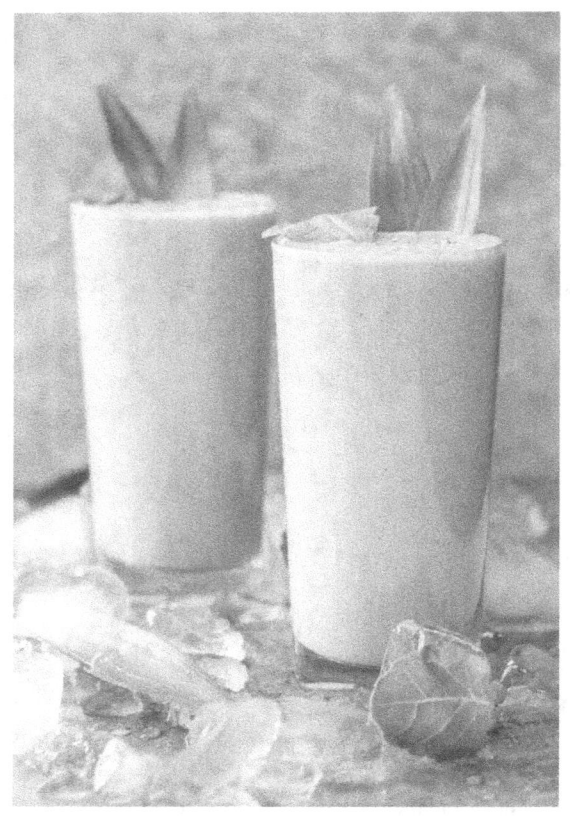

INGREDIENTS:

Green apple – 1 piece
Cucumber – 1 piece
Chopped pineapple – 100 gr
Kale leaves – 4 pcs
Swiss Chard leaves – 3 pcs

DIRECTIONS:

1. Wash, peel (if necessary) and chop all ingredients.
2. Put all ingredients in your juicer and make a fresh green juice.

5. Deep Green Juice

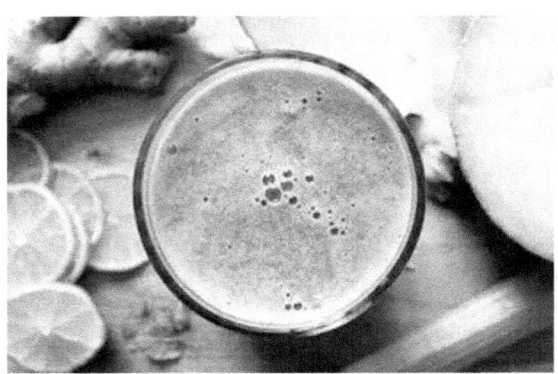

INGREDIENTS:

Green apple – 2 pcs
Cucumber – 1 piece
Collard leaves – 6 pcs
Celery ribs - 2 pcs
Half of 1 lemon
Fennel bulbs - ⅛

DIRECTIONS:

1. Wash, peel (if necessary) and chop all ingredients.
2. Put them in your juicer and make a juice.

6. Clean Green

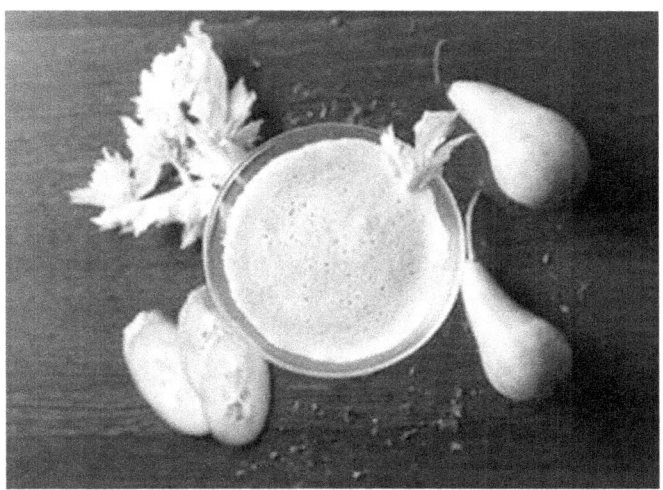

INGREDIENTS:

Pears – 3 pcs
Zucchini – 1 piece
Fennel bulb - ⅛
Broccoli florets – 4 pcs
Spinach one bunch

DIRECTIONS:

1. Wash, peel (if necessary) and chop all ingredients.
2. Put them in your juicer and make a juice.

7. Green Detox

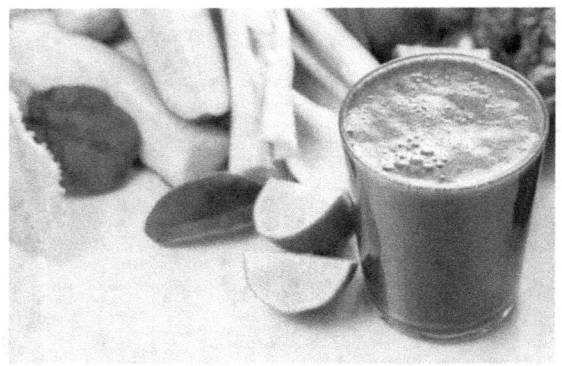

INGREDIENTS:

Cilantro – one bunch
Cucumbers – 2 pcs
Green apple – 2 pcs
Lime – 1 piece

DIRECTIONS:

1. Wash, peel (if necessary) and chop all ingredients.
2. Put them in your juicer and make a juice.

8. Pineapple Mint

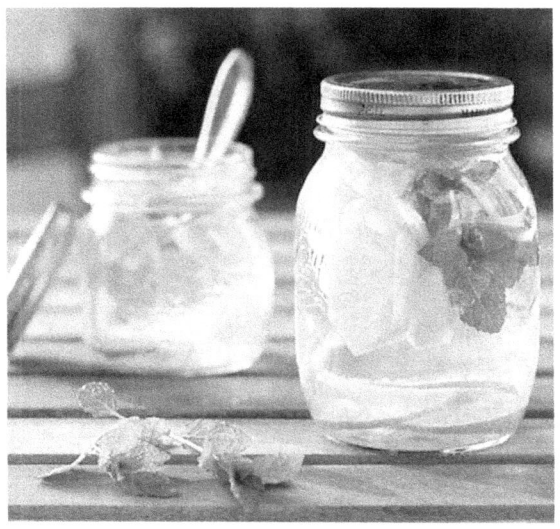

INGREDIENTS:

Chopped pineapple – one cup
Mint leaves (chopped) – 30 g
Green apple – 2 pcs
Spinach (chopped) - 60 g
Kale leaves – 4 pcs

DIRECTIONS:

1. Wash, peel (if necessary) and chop all ingredients.
2. Put them in your juicer and make a juice.

9. Glow Juice

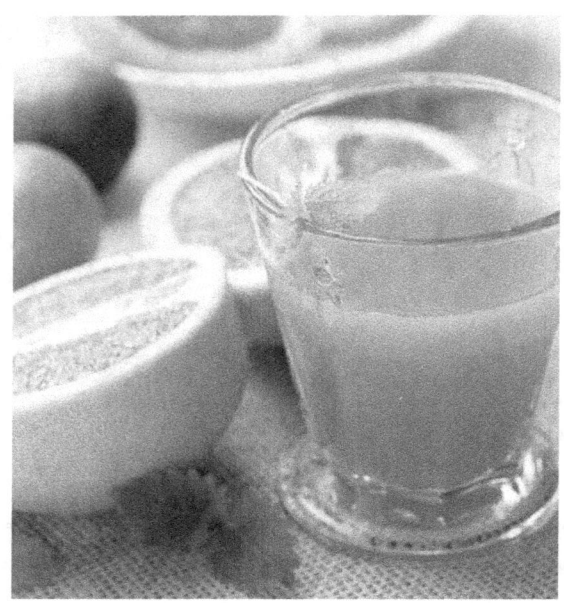

INGREDIENTS:

Grapefruit – 2 pcs
Cucumber – 2 pcs Basil – five-six sprigs
Mint leaves (chopped) – 2 pcs
Coconut Sugar – 10 gr
Cantaloupe - ¼

DIRECTIONS:

1. Wash, peel (if necessary) and chop all ingredients.
2. Put them in your juicer and make a juice.

10. Soothing Juice

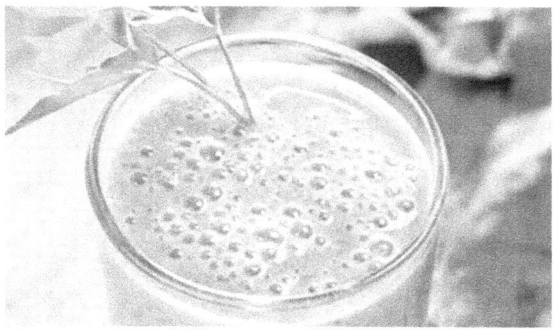

INGREDIENTS:

Green apple – 2 pcs
Cucumber – 2 pcs
Lemon – 1 piece
Honey – 50 gr
Ginger - ½ inch

DIRECTIONS:

1. Wash, peel (if necessary) and chop all ingredients.
2. Put them in your juicer and make a juice.

11. Anti-Allergy Juice

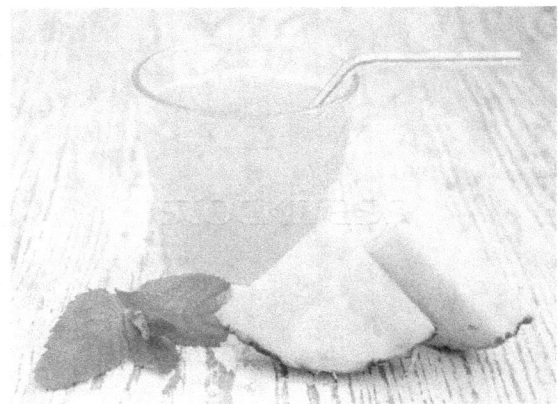

INGREDIENTS:

Pineapple (chopped) 200 gr
Lemon – 2 pcs
Cucumber – 1 piece
Parsley (chopped) – 70 gr
Apple – 1 piece
Ginger – one inch

DIRECTIONS:

1. Wash, peel (if necessary) and chop all ingredients.
2. Put them in your juicer and make a juice.

12. Mango & Kale Juice

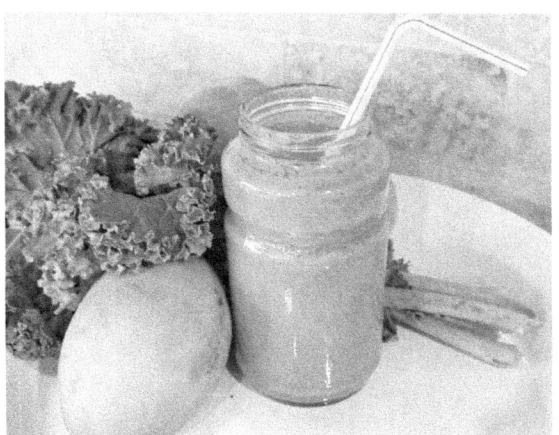

INGREDIENTS:

Mango – 1 piece
Kale leaves (chopped) – 150 g
Spinach (chopped) – 150 gr
Apple – 1 piece
Coconut water - 120 ml

DIRECTIONS:

1. Wash, peel (if necessary) and chop all ingredients.
2. Put them in your juicer and make a juice.

13. Spinach Lemonade

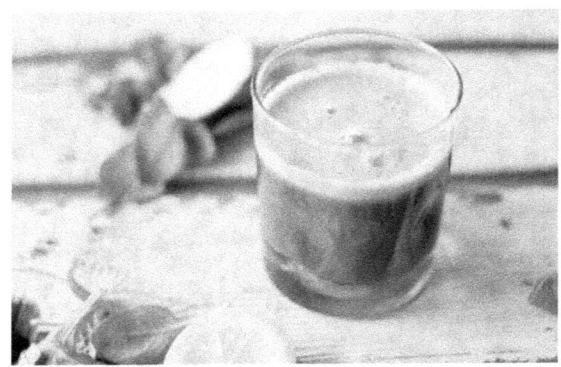

INGREDIENTS:

Spinach (chopped) – 700 gr
Lemon – 2 pcs
Half of 1 cucumber
Pear – one piece
Green Apple – 2 pcs

DIRECTIONS:

1. Wash, peel (if necessary) and chop all ingredients.
2. Put them in your juicer and make a spinach lemonade.

14. Lettuce Juice

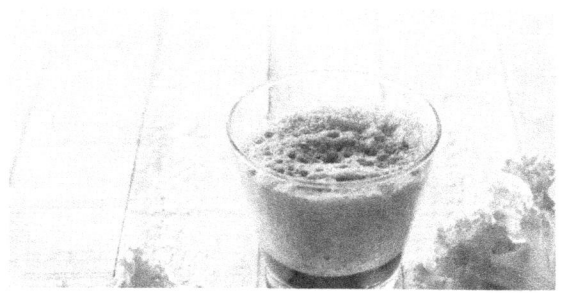

INGREDIENTS:

Romaine lettuce – one head
Celery - 2 pcs
Kale – five stalks
Apple – 2 pcs
Lemon – one piece
Ginger – 25-30 g
Watercress - ½ bunch
Cayenne Pepper (to taste)

DIRECTIONS:

1. Wash, peel (if necessary) and chop all ingredients.
2. Put them in your juicer and make a juice.

15. Basil - Cucumber Juice

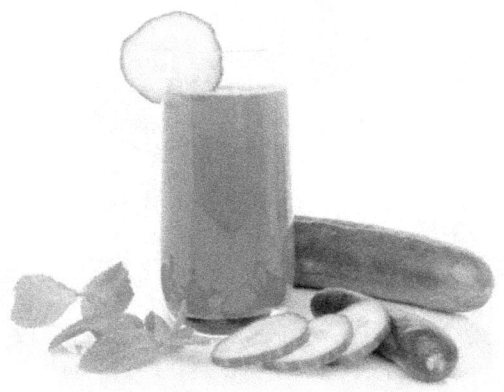

INGREDIENTS:

Basil (chopped) 60 g
Apple – 2 pcs
Cucumber – 1 piece
Lime – 1 piece

DIRECTIONS:

1. Wash, peel (if necessary) and chop all ingredients.
2. Put them in your juicer and make a juice.

16. Kale Kiwi Juice

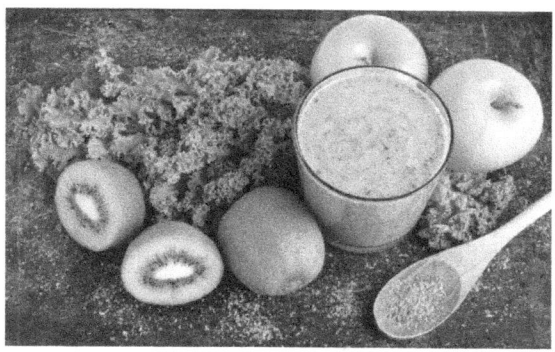

INGREDIENTS:

Kale – one bunch
Kiwi – 3 pcs
Apple – 2 pcs
Ginger: 1 inch

DIRECTIONS:

1. Wash, peel (if necessary) and chop all ingredients.
2. Put them in your juicer and make a juice.

17. "Silly monkeys" Smoothie

(4 servings)

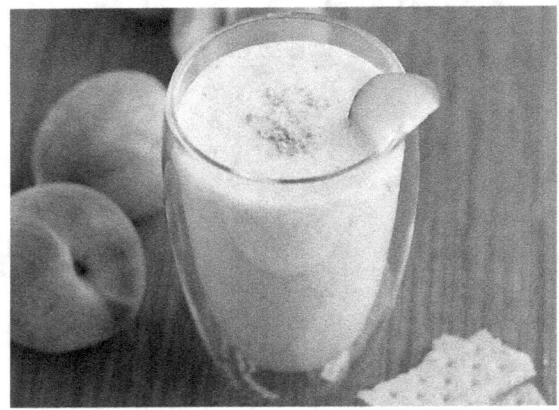

INGREDIENTS:

Frozen bananas – 3 pcs
Sunflower butter – 60 g
Apple juice – 120 ml
"Safe" milk – 180 ml

DIRECTIONS:

1) Soften the bananas and slice them.
2) Put all ingredients in your blender and make a fresh smoothie.
3) Serve immediately!

NUTRITION: 167 calories; 28 g carbohydrates; 5 gr protein; 4 g fiber; 5 g total fat; 0.7 g saturated fat.

18. Pineapple and Spirulina Smoothie

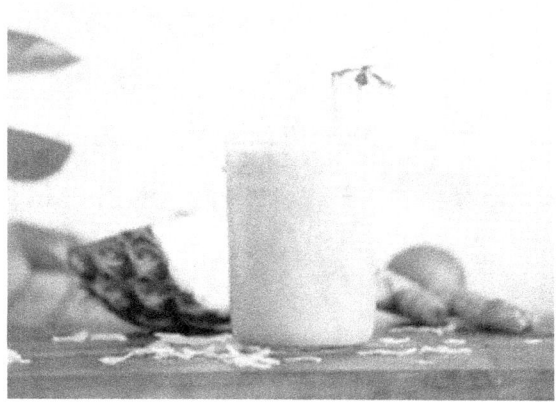

INGREDIENTS:

Pineapple – 300 gr
Spirulina powder – 5 gr

DIRECTIONS:

1. Wash, peel (if necessary) and chop all ingredients.
2. Put them in your juicer and make fresh smoothie.

19. Broccoli and Spinach Smoothie

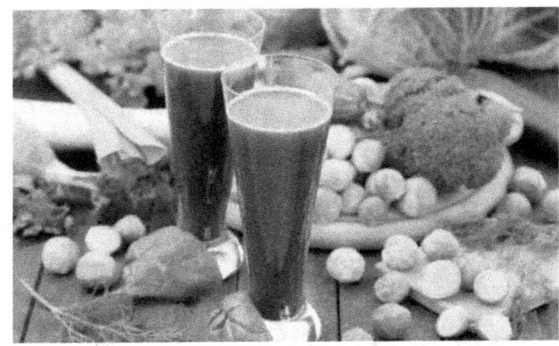

INGREDIENTS:

Broccoli (chopped) – 150 gr
Spinach (chopped) – 120 gr
Kale leaves – 2 pcs
Half of one green apple
Half of one cucumber
Half of one avocado
Fresh juice of one lime

DIRECTIONS:

1. Wash, peel (if necessary) and chop all ingredients.
2. Put all ingredients in your blender and make a fresh smoothie.

20. Allergy Cure Juice Recipe

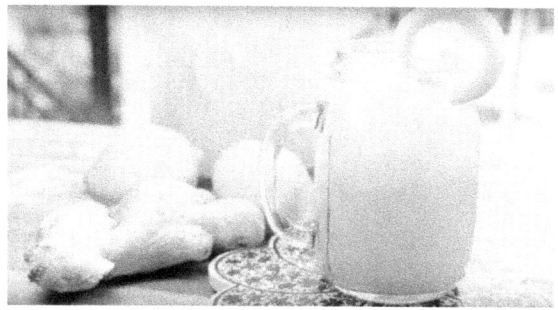

INGREDIENTS:

Ginger – 1 knob
Lemon – 1 piece
Garlic bulbets – 3 pcs
Cucumber – 1 piece

DIRECTIONS:

1. Wash, peel (if necessary) and chop all ingredients.
2. Put all ingredients in your vegetable juicer.
3. Sprinkle with finely chopped parsley. Enjoy immediately!

21. Anti-Allergy Smoothie

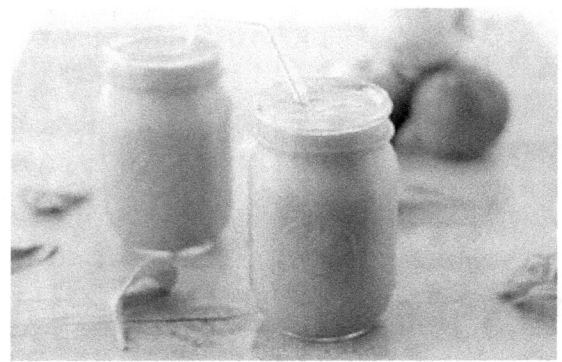

INGREDIENTS:

Sliced cantaloupe – 2 pcs
Ginger root -1/4 inch
Half of one apple
Green powder – 10 g

DIRECTIONS:

1. Wash, peel (if necessary) and chop all ingredients.
2. Put all ingredients in your blender and make a fresh smoothie.

RECIPES OF ANTI-ALLERGY SOUPS

22. Sweet Potato Soup with Thyme (6-8 servings)

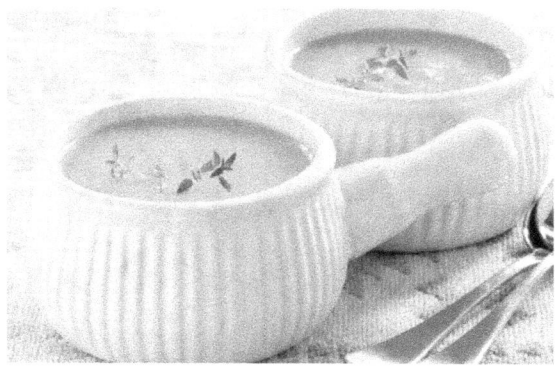

INGREDIENTS:

Vegetable broth – 1500 ml
Large sweet potatoes - 3 pcs
Yellow onion – 2 pcs
Fresh ginger - 1/2 inch
Olive oil – 18 g
Fresh thyme
Salt and pepper

DIRECTIONS:

1. Wash, peel and chop potatoes, onion and ginger.
2. Heat olive oil in a saucepan. Add chopped onion and fry on a medium heat until golden brown
3. Then pour vegetable broth and bring to boil. Add chopped sweet potatoes and ginger. Let it boil on a medium heat.
4. Cook about 20 to 25 minutes.
5. Purée soup, add salt, pepper, fresh thyme to taste.
6. Serve hot!

23. Chicken Noodle Soup

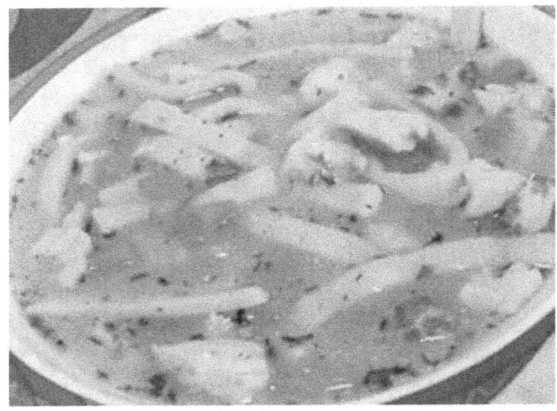

INGREDIENTS:

Chicken broth – 1500 ml (gluten free)
Frozen mixed vegetables – 160 gr
Gluten free brown rice spiral pasta – 150 gr
Cooked chicken – 250 g, chopped
Onion – 1 piece, chopped
Garlic bulbet – 1 piece, minced
Celery stalks – 2 pcs, chopped
Carrot – 1 piece, chopped
Petite cut tomatoes – one can (14.5 ounce)
Salt and pepper
Dried oregano leaves – 5 g
Dried basil leaves – 5 g
Bay leaf – 1 piece

DIRECTIONS:

1. Chop cooked chicken, onion, garlic, carrot and celery stalks.
2. Take a deep saucepan and pour there chicken broth, add spices, onion, garlic, chopped celery stalks, carrot and frozen mixed vegetables.
3. Bring it to a boil. Cook 7-10 minutes, then add gluten free brown rice spiral pasta. Let it cook for 12-15 minutes.
4. Add tomatoes and cooked chicken. Cook for another 5 minutes. Add salt and pepper to taste.
5. Bon appetite!

RECIPES OF ANTI-ALLERGY SNACKS, BREAKFASTS and DINNERS

24. Turkey Breakfast Sausage

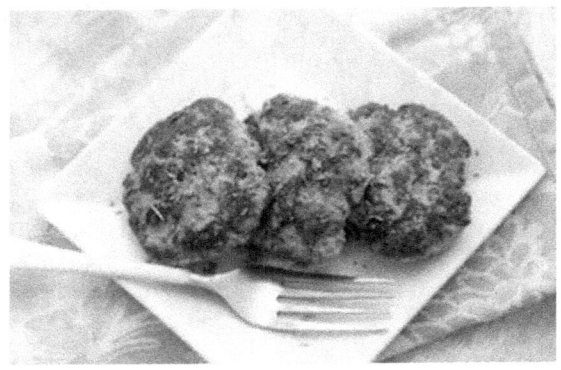

INGREDIENTS:

Extra virgin olive oil – 5 gr
Onion – 1 piece
Garlic bulbet – 1piece
Ground turkey 900 gr
Fennel seed – 50-60 gr
Rubbed sage – two tsp
Salt – 5-10 gr
Pepper – 5 gr
Red pepper flakes
"Safe" cooking spray

DIRECTIONS:

1. Peel and chop onion, mince garlic.
2. Take a pan and pour olive oil. Add the finely chopped onion and minced garlic and fry until cooked. Then let it cool.
3. Take a bowl and combine all of the remaining ingredients. Add fried onion and garlic mixture. Stir together.
4. Make turkey burgers.

5. Take a pan, spray some cooking spray. Fry the burgers on both sides.

6. Your turkey patties are ready. Enjoy hot or cool.

NUTRITION: Serving Size: 1 patty, 113 calories; 55 fat calories; 1 g carbohydrates; 12 gr protein; 4 g fiber; 6 g total fat; 1.5 g saturated fat.

25. Cottage Cheese Casserole

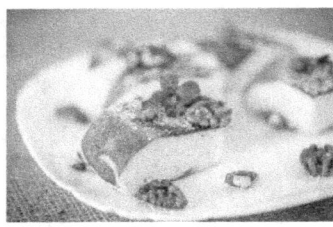

INGREDIENTS:

Low-fat cottage cheese 180 g
Chicken egg - 1 piece (if you don't avoid eggs)
Apple (chopped) - 50 g
Oat bran – 12 gr.
Yogurt -30 gr

DIRECTIONS:

1. Mash cheese.
2. Add 12 gr of oat bran and 50 gr of finely chopped apple. Add one egg. Mix thoroughly.
3. Grease baking dish with yogurt. Transfer cheese mass into the dish.
4. Cook at 190 degrees for 20-25 minutes.

26. Crunchy Coleslaw Recipe

(12 servings)

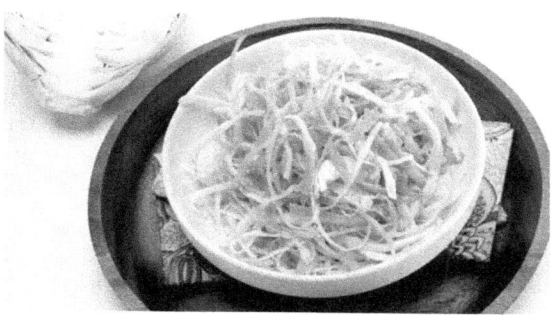

INGREDIENTS:

Shredded coleslaw mix – 1 package (16 oz.)
Granny Smith apple (diced) – 3 cups
Seedless raisins
Plain "safe" yogurt (soy or coconut) - 1/3 cup
Canola mayonnaise – 3 tbsp
Honey – 2 tbsp
Granulated sugar – 1 tbsp
Pepper – 0,5 tsp
Salt – 1 tsp

DIRECTIONS:

1. Take two bowls.
2. Put 1 package of shredded coleslaw mix, diced apples and seedless raisins in one bowl. Mix together.
3. Take another bowl and make a sauce. Put there 1/3 cup of yogurt, 3 tablespoons of mayonnaise, 2 tablespoons of honey, salt and pepper. Mix carefully.
4. Pour this sauce over coleslaw mixture and toss well. Let it cool.
5. Serve and enjoy!

NUTRITION: Serving Size: 1/2 cup, 73 calories; 15 g carbohydrates; 1.1 gr protein; 1.8 g fiber; 1 g total fat; 0.1 g saturated fat.

27. Chili

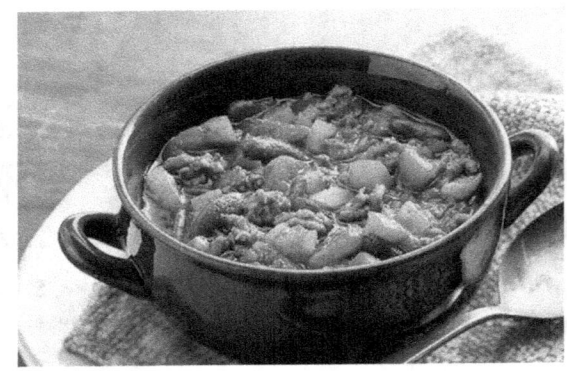

INGREDIENTS:

Lean ground beef – 450 gr
Beef broth – 240 ml
Diced tomatoes – 2x14.5oz cans
Dark red kidney beans – 2x16oz. can
Black beans – 1x15 oz. can
Tomato sauce – 1x 8oz. can
Onion – 1 piece
Garlic bulbet – 1
Celery -1 stalk
Salt – 5 gr
Pepper – 2.5 gr
Ground cumin – 10 gr
Chili powder – 30 gr
Bay leaf – 1 piece

DIRECTIONS:

1) Prepare ingredients before you start cooking. Chop onion and celery stalk. Mince garlic bulbet. Drain beans.
2) Take a stockpot and lightly brown the hamburger. Drain fat.
3) Add chopped onion, minced garlic and chopped celery stalks. Cook until tender.

4) Salt and pepper to taste and pour beef broth. Add diced tomatoes with juice, tomato sauce and some water, drained kidney beans and black beans, one bay leaf and spices. Stir slowly all ingredients. Bring to boil, slack the fire and stew for about one hour.

5) Better taste with corn tortilla chips.

6) Make 14 cups.

NUTRITION: Serving Size: 1 cup, 196 calories; 74 fat calories; 19 g carbohydrates; 11.4 gr protein; 7.5 g fiber; 8.5 g total fat; 3.4 g saturated fat.

28. Allergy Free Chicken Pot Pies

(Makes 4 servings)

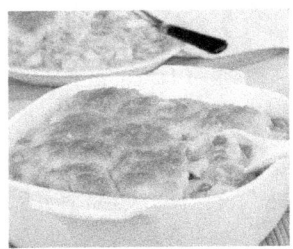

INGREDIENTS:

Gluten-free pie crust – 1
Cooking spray
White rice flour – 120 gr
Rubbed sage - 10 gr
Chicken breasts – 450 gr
"Safe" margarine – 40 gr
"Safe" milk – 240 ml
Gluten-free chicken broth – 60 ml
Water – 300 ml
Frozen vegetable mixture - 1,5 cup
Mushrooms – 225 gr
Black pepper
Salt
Buy beforehand gluten-free ready-made pie crusts!

DIRECTIONS:

1) First of all, let`s prepare the toppers for the pie crust:
2) Preheat the oven to 220 C. Take a dough and cut out four 3-4 inch circles.
3) Place them on a baking sheet greased with cooking spray. Coat your circles with cooking spray too and drizzle with salt. Pierce the top of circles with a fork.
4) Bake at 220 C for 8 minutes.
5) Now, it`s time to make a sauce. Melt the margarine a saucepan.
6) Add 120 gr of white rice flour, then stir together.
7) Pour 240 ml of milk and 60 ml of chicken broth. Stir again. Cook until thickened.

8) Take a chicken, chop into pieces. Prepare a mixture of sage, flour, salt, pepper and flour. Cover chicken with this mixture.

9) Take a pan, add some cooking spray and heat it. Put the chicken and lightly brown on all sides.

10) Add some water, frozen vegetable mixture, mushrooms and sauce. Bring to boil.

11) Stew for about 10 minutes.

12) Top with one pie crust round.

NUTRITION: Serving Size: 1 cup, 440 calories; 187 fat calories; 26 g carbohydrates; 36 gr protein; 4 g fiber; 21 g total fat; 4 g saturated fat.

29. Red Beans and Rice Skillet

(8 servings)

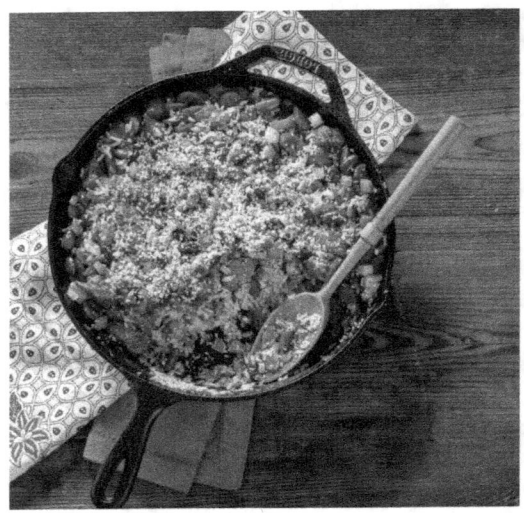

INGREDIENTS:

Turkey kielbasa – 400 g
Yellow onion – 1 piece
Green bell pepper – 1 piece
Garlic bulbet – 1 piece
Dark red kidney beans – 2x16 oz. cans
Italian style diced tomatoes – 1x14,5 oz. can
Uncooked rice - 1/2 cup
Pepper – 0,5 tsp.
Cooking spray
Water – 240 ml

DIRECTIONS:

1) Peel and chop onion and mince garlic. Drain dark red kidney beans. Slice turkey kielbasa diagonally in 1/4 inch pieces.
2) Take a pan and spray it with cooking spray. Fry the sausage on low heat for about 5 minutes.

3) Add chopped onion, green bell pepper and minced garlic. Fry until onion golden brown. Put drained beans, a can of tomatoes and some pepper. Cook10-15 minutes.
4) Pour 240 ml of water, rice and mix. Bring to boil, cover the pan and stew for 20 minutes.
5) Enjoy hot!

NUTRITION: Serving Size: 1 cup, 205 calories; 187 fat calories; 27 g carbohydrates; 16 gr protein; 8.5 g fiber; 4.4 g total fat.

30. Quinoa and Rice with Sweet Potatoes

(6 servings)

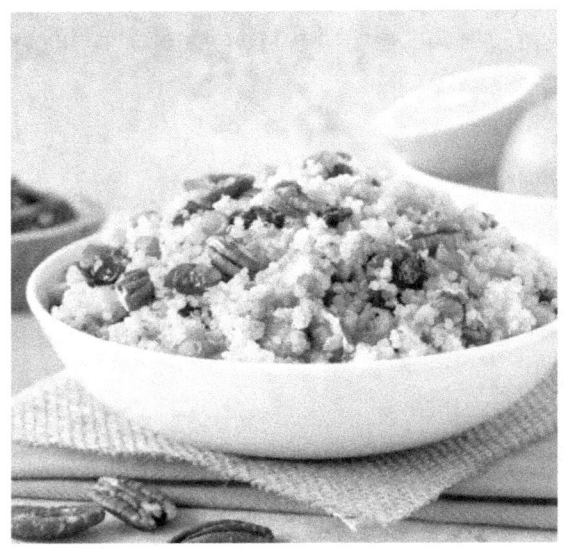

INGREDIENTS:

"Safe" cooking spray
Extra virgin olive oil 18 gr
Onion – 1 piece
Carrot – 1 piece
Celery – 3 stalks
Sweet potato 1 piece
Uncooked brown rice – 145 gr
Uncooked quinoa - 3/4 cup
"safe" low sodium vegetable or chicken broth – 700 ml
Sea salt – 10 gr

DIRECTIONS:

1. Preheat the oven to 180° C. Take a casserole dish and spray with cooking spray

2. Take a pan, pour the olive oil and fry finely chopped onion, carrot and celery , peeled and chopped sweet potato. Fry until cooked.
3. Add brown rice, uncooked quinoa, broth and 10 gr of sea salt to the vegetable mixture. Pour this mixture into the greased casserole; cover and cook for about 30-40 minutes.

NUTRITION: Serving Size: 1 cup, 237 calories; 42 g carbohydrates; 7.7 gr protein; 4.2 g fiber; fat: 4.8 g

ANTI-ALLERGY DESSERTS

31. Banana Boats

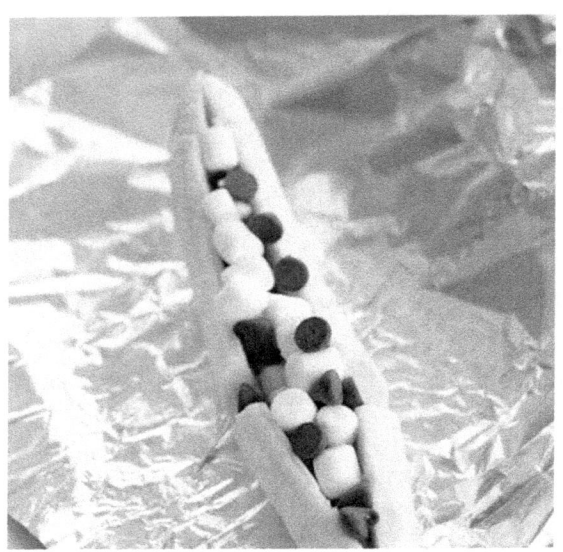

INGREDIENTS:

Banana – 1 piece
Sunflower butter – 0,5 tbsp
"Safe" semi-sweet chocolate chips – 2 tsp
"Safe" mini marshmallows – 2 tbsp

DIRECTIONS:

1. This dish may be prepared on the campfire or grill
2. Peel one strip from the banana.
3. Cut banana into circles.
4. Take an aluminum foil and place sunflower butter. Then put the chocolate chips, mini marshmallows on top of the sunflower butter. Then put banana circles.
5. Wrap in aluminum foil and grill for 5-10 minutes.

6. Unfold the foil and place grilled bananas on the skin.

NUTRITION: Serving Size: 1 banana boat, 220 calories; 60 fat calories; 39 g carbohydrates; 3.5 gr protein; 4.5 g fiber; 7 g total fat; 2 g saturated fat.

32. Allergy Free Birthday Cake

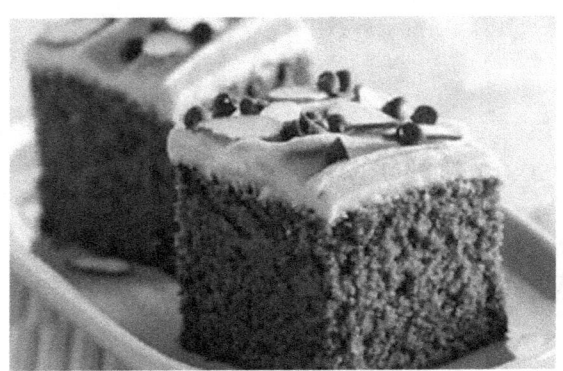

INGREDIENTS:

White rice flour - 140 gr
Potato starch (not potato flour) – 47 gr
Tapioca starch – 90 gr
Xanthan gum – 0,5 tsp
Sugar - 190 gr
Cocoa powder – 35 gr
Salt – 5 gr
Baking soda – 10 gr
Pure vanilla extract – 10 gr
Vinegar (any you like) – 20 gr
Canola oil – 90 gr
Cold water – 175ml

DIRECTIONS:

1. Preheat the oven to 180 C.
2. Take a bowl and put there potato starch, cocoa powder, rice flour, tapioca starch, sugar, some salt, xanthan gum, and baking soda. Mix all ingredients.
3. Add pure vanilla extract, 20 gr of vinegar, 90 gr of canola oil and water. Mix thoroughly.
4. Take a square cake pan. Don`t grease it. Pour batter into it. Cook at 180 degrees for half an hour.

For cupcakes: Pour batter into a muffin form with paper liners. Turn on the oven and heat it to 180 C. Bake for half an hour. Remove your ready cake immediately. Cut it into 12 cupcakes.

NUTRITION: Serving Size: 1 cupcake, 165 calories; 54 fat calories; 28 g carbohydrates; 1.5 gr protein; 1 g fiber; 6 g total fat; 0.6 g saturated fat.

33. Fruit Buckle

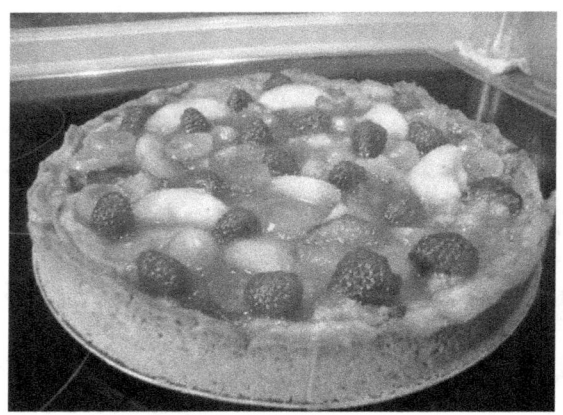

INGREDIENTS:

Gluten-free flour mix - 1,5cups
No milk margarine - 1/4 cup
Nondairy milk - 1,5 cups
Sugar - 1,5 cups
Xanthan gum - 0,5 tsp
White vinegar – 36 gr
Fresh or frozen fruits - 2 cups
Baking powder - 20 gr
Granulated sugar – 60 gr
Salt – 0,5 tsp

DIRECTIONS:

1) Turn on the oven and preheat it to 180 C. Put margarine into the pan and melt it.
2) Take a bowl. Combine dry ingredients (60 gr of sugar,1,5 cups of the flour, 0,5 tsp of xanthan gum, 20 gr of baking powder, some salt). Make a batter.
3) Pour it into the pan. Put fruits on the top. Drizzle with sugar.
4) Bake for about one hour.
5) Enjoy warm with allergy free ice cream.

NUTRITION: Serving Size: for 1 piece, 170 calories; 33.3 fat calories; 33 g carbohydrates; 2.4 gr protein; 1.4 g fiber; 3.7 g total fat; 0.5 g saturated fat.

34. Nut Free Granola Bars

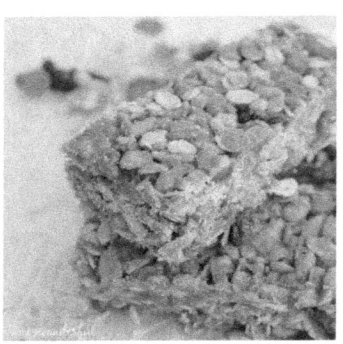

INGREDIENTS:

Brown sugar – 125 gr
Canola oil – 80 gr
Molasses – two tbsp
Water – 60 ml
Flax seed meal - 1/3 cup
Sunflower butter - 2/3 cup
Protein powder - 1/4 cup
Sunflower seed - 1/3 cup
Oatmeal- 3 cups
Salt – 2 gr
Vanilla – 10 gr

DIRECTIONS:

1) Preheat the oven to 180 C in advance. Take a pan and spray it with cooking spray.
2) Take a bowl and mix oil and molasses, brown sugar in it; add vanilla, some salt, sunflower butter, water, flax seed meal, protein powder and mix again.
3) Then add the oats and sunflower seeds. Pour batter into the baking pan.
4) Bake in preheated oven for 18-20 minutes. Remove your dish from the oven and let it cool completely.
5) Take a knife and cut into squared portions.

NUTRITION: Serving Size: 1 bar, 144 calories; 17 g carbohydrates; 6 gr protein; 3 g fiber; 6 g total fat.

Top Seventeen Best and Anti-Allergy Foods

1. Apples (contain quercetin, a flavonoid which may protect against allergic reactions, improve immune system).
2. Rose Hips (it is one of the best natural anti-allergy products. Enriched with vitamins E and C).
3. Turmeric (it is powerful antioxidant. Contains curcumin and anti-inflammatory compounds).
4. Rosemary (It contains rosmarinic acid, that suppresses allergic reactions).
5. Lemon (it is the best natural anti-allergy food. Lemon is the source of antioxidants and vitamin C. This fruit strengthens immune system).
6. Garlic (it is the best natural anti-allergy food. It contains compounds that prevent allergic reactions. It has antioxidant, anti-inflammatory, immune-boosting, antibiotic properties).
7. Dandelion Greens (it contains vitamins E and C, beta-carotene. It helps to treat allergy).
8. Salmon (anti-allergy food, it is enriched with Omega-3 fatty acids).
9. Mushrooms (this food can alleviate allergic reactions. It contains selenium).
10. Green Tea (it boosts up immune system and prevents allergy reactions. It has anti-histamine, anti-inflammatory, antioxidant properties).
11. Mustard Greens (it is full of nutrients and antioxidants, vitamins C, E).
12. Sweet Potatoes (it is a source of potassium, beta-carotene, contains manganese, vitamin. It reduces inflammation).
13. Sunflower Seeds (Seeds has fat and calories. It is a great source of vitamin E and selenium).
14. Ginger (it has great antioxidant and anti-inflammatory effect).
15. Anchovies (this fish is high in selenium and Omega-3 fatty acids).
16. Collard Greens (contain phytochemicals (carotenoids). It helps to prevent allergy).
17. Flaxseeds (Has selenium, Omega-3 fatty acids and. It helps to prevent allergy. Improve immune system).

Thank You

I am very happy that you have chosen this book and it's been a real pleasure writing it for you. My aim is to help as many readers as possible. So many of us are able to take new knowledge and use it to our lives with really useful and long lasting consequences and it is my desire that you have been able to take value from the information I have written.

Thank you for being with me during this book and for reading it through to the end. I really hope that you have enjoyed the information and that's why I appreciate your thoughts on my material so much. If you could take a couple of minutes to write a feedback, your views will help me to create more material that you find beneficial.

Thanks again for your attention. I really look forward to reading your review.

Stay Healthy!

BY THE SAME AUTHOR

You are welcome to read another useful and very informative books which are written by me!

PALEO DIET FOR BEGINNERS

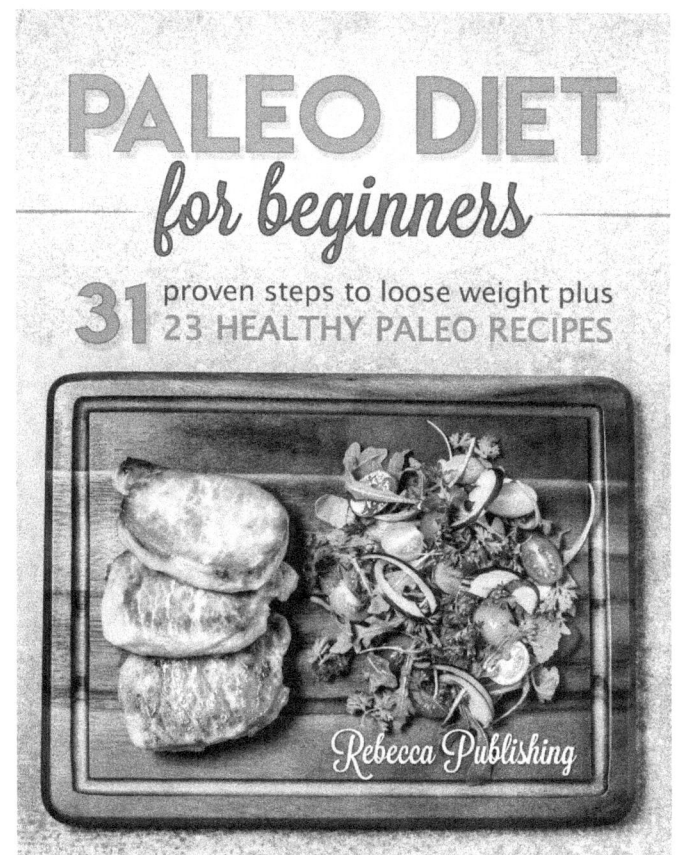

Please search this page over the www.amazon.com

www.amazon.com/s/ref=nb_sb_noss_2?url=search-alias%3Daps&field-keywords=B01MR9UU2O

KETOGENIC DIET FOR BEGINNERS

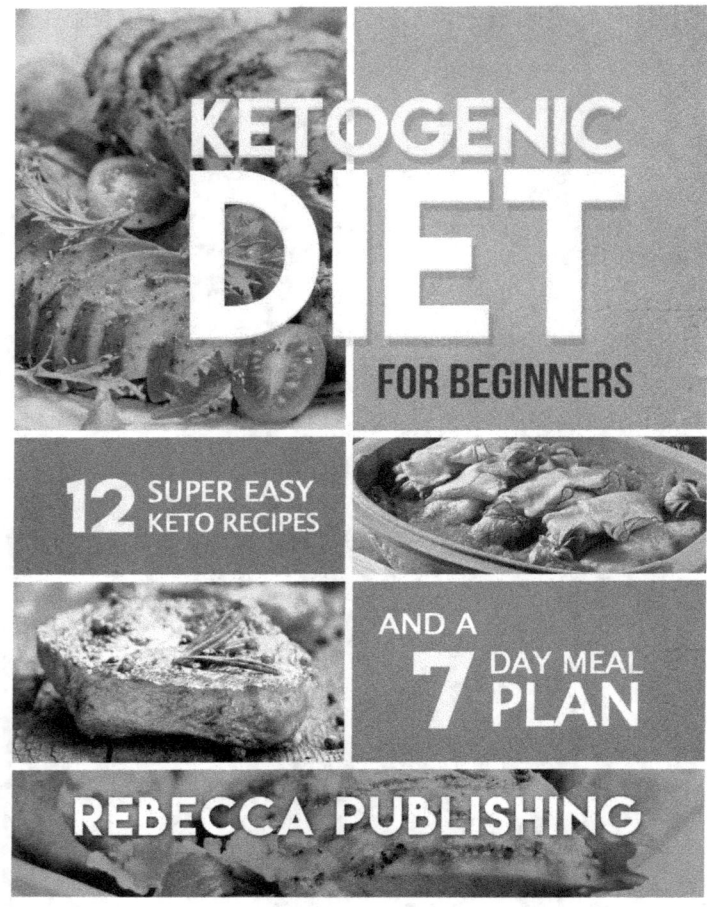

Please search this page over the www.amazon.com

www.amazon.com/s/ref=nb_sb_noss_2?url=search-alias%3Daps&field-keywords=1544626592

ANTI-INFLAMMATORY DIET

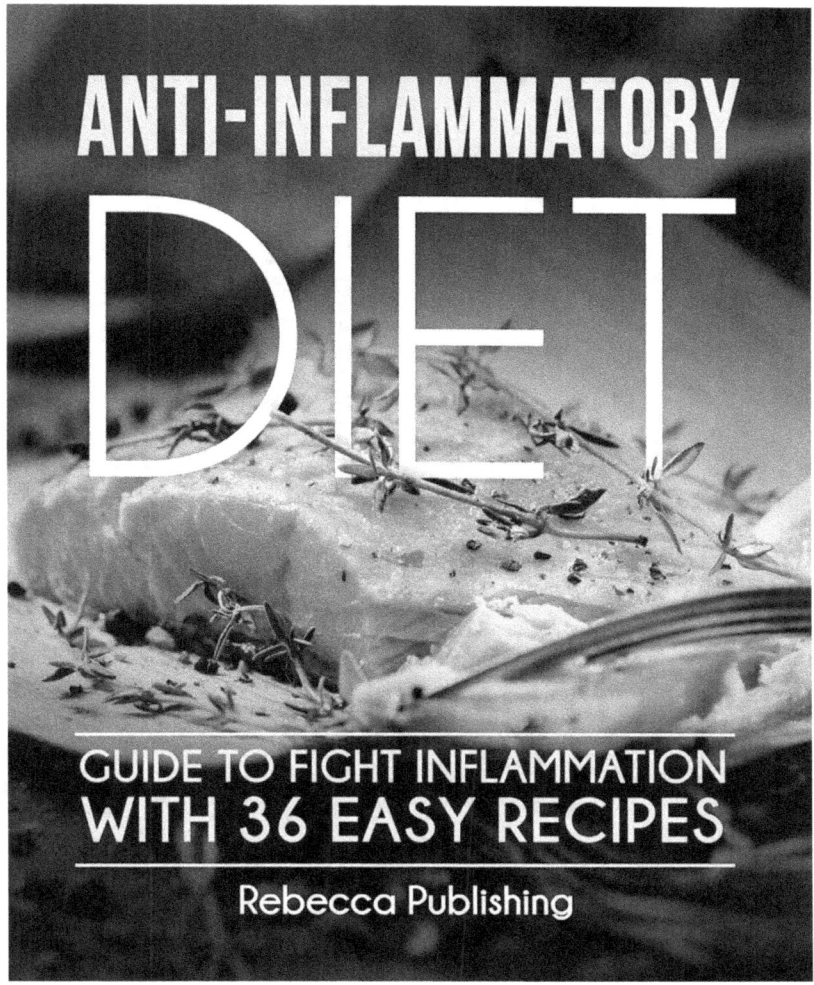

Please search this page over the www.amazon.com

www.amazon.com/s/ref=nb_sb_noss?url=search-alias%3Daps&field-keywords=B0718WKD81

35 PALEO AND KET RECIPES

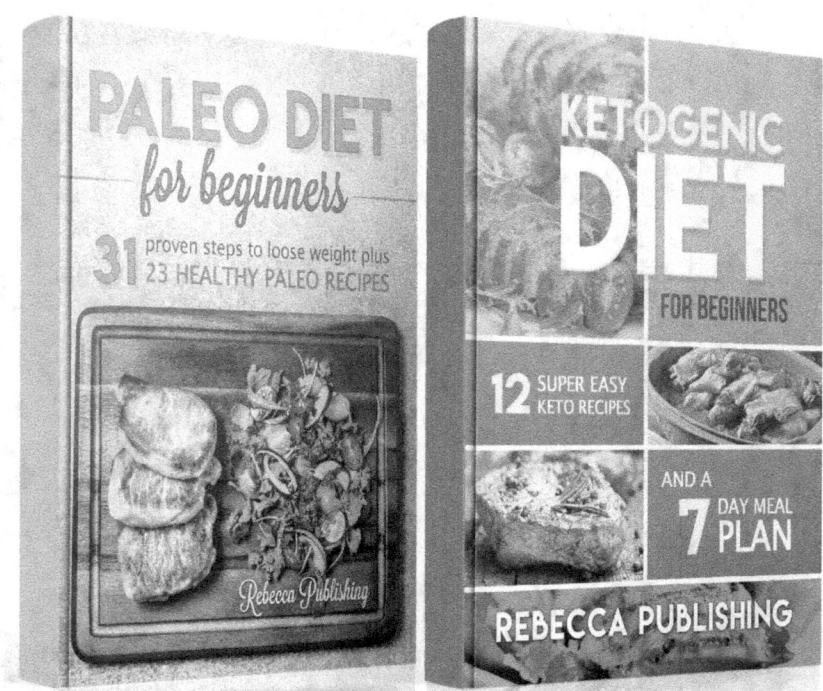